Other Books by the Author

Pediatrics: Some Uncommon Views on Some
Common Problems

Professionally Speaking: Public Speaking for Health
Professionals

Medical Writing 101

A Primer for Health Professionals

by

Arnold Melnick, DO, MSc,
DHL (Hon.), FACOP

Trine University
Health Education Center - FWRC
1819 Carew Street
Fort Wayne, IN 46805

Bloomington, IN Milton Keynes, UK

authorHOUSE

AuthorHouse™
1663 Liberty Drive, Suite 200
Bloomington, IN 47403
www.authorhouse.com
Phone: 1-800-839-8640

AuthorHouse™ UK Ltd.
500 Avebury Boulevard
Central Milton Keynes, MK9 2BE
www.authorhouse.co.uk
Phone: 08001974150

First published by AuthorHouse 3/30/2006

  ISBN: 1-4259-1281-8 (sc)

Library of Congress Control Number: 2006900046

Printed in the United States of America
Bloomington, Indiana

This book is printed on acid-free paper.

Medical Writing 101:

A Primer for Health Professionals

DEDICATION

Forever
to my wonderful wife
Anita
my most ardent critic and support
I love you!

CONTENTS

Acknowledgements

I have been privileged to learn about writing, and medical writing, from hundreds of persons, from my first Sunday School teacher to whatever medical writer I most recently happened to speak to. Each deserves from a paragraph to a page for proper acknowledgement, and I wish I had space for it. Alas, I have not.

I have learned from all of them. I also feel I have borrowed unconsciously from all of them. I hope I have included all my benefactors and gratefully I recognize my debt to them for a life full of enjoyable writing.

Katherine Becker
Francis DiPiano, Ph.D.
Harold H. Finkel, D.O.
Ray Hulburt, D.O.
Raymond Keesecker, D.O.
Julian Mines, D.O.
Barbara Peterson
Charles G. Roland, M.D.
Milton J. Schiffrin, Ph.D.

Edith Schwager
George F. Stickley
Irving J. Wolman, M.D.

Plus hundreds of other students, colleagues, various editors, and members of the American Medical Writers Association, for thousands of ideas and suggestions over the years.

Preface

The mission of medical writing, indeed all kinds of writing, is COMMUNICATION! One writes (or speaks) and others are expected to understand. Principles and rules should, for the most part, help us with that goal, but should never get in the way of communicating and thinking.

Most readers will immediately recognize that Medical Writing 101 means an introductory course, starting with the basics and covering the fundamentals of the subject. For beginners, this book should provide an insight into various aspects of medical writing. Some beginners may already know some of the introductory principles, while others may know different aspects. My hope is that this book will provide a strong training program for all in basic medical writing, teach some new topics and refresh the reader's knowledge of other areas.

Those with writing experience will know a great deal about the principles but this book should provide a refresher for them and maybe add a few new ideas in medical writing.

This book, of course, can be used as the text for an organized course in medical writing. Since there are very few such courses, it can also serve well as a self-training manual and an on-going reference. This is truly a primer, written to explain from the simplest basics to the more intricate without becoming too complicated. The book is devised so that it can actually serve as a tutorial.

A word needs to be said about whom we have in mind with the words "medical writing." In this book, the reader will be addressed as physician or medical student. However, the book is directed at *all* health professionals because in the realm of medical writing all health professionals are equal—whether dentists, optometrists, nurses, podiatrists, pharmacists, allied health personnel or any others in the field. Students of all the professions are included in the term medical students. Almost all of us in the health fields can use help when it comes to medical writing. This book is not meant, however, to be the reverse -- a text of medical information for writers seeking to enter the field of medical writing, and needing medical background.

To the successful writers in the health professions and to those who by training or experience can write adequately — that's not everybody — my congratulations. But even you may want to take a look occasionally into a help book like this.

To all readers, remember that every published author, whether medical writer, novelist, poet or whatever, has been backed by a strong editor. This is the key to successful publication. None of us is above needing a good editor. I hope there will be something here for everybody.

So, welcome and good luck in your medical writing.

Introduction to Medical Writing

In promulgating your esoteric cogitations or articulating your superficial or philosophic sentimentalities, beware of platitudinous ponderosities. Let your conversational communications possess a clarified conciseness and compacted comprehensiveness. Eschew all conglomerations of flatulent garrulities.

I use that little paragraph as my opening in everything I teach in medical writing, whether it is a course or simply a single lecture. I use it because it illustrates succinctly, and hopefully humorously, one of the most important points in medical writing. I do not use any introduction to it, but immediately upon presenting it, I explain its meaning: don't use big words, talk plainly.

That message leads me directly into explaining why doctors need to know about medical writing.

In the first few courses that I taught to medical students, I would follow that little recital with a question to the class, "How many of you expect to do any medical writing?"

Generally, I would get one or two hands raised. This would be my springboard to a sermonette about the reasons physicians need to be able to do medical writing. However, as in so many instances, the students taught the instructor a trick. At the suggestion of several students in my first couple of classes, I changed my follow-up. I eliminated the preaching. When only one or two hands went up in response to my initial question, I would then ask, "How many of you ever expect to write a medical article?" Again, I would get the same one or two hands. Without showing any discouragement, I would then ask "How many of you expect to write patient notes on hospital or office charts?" More hands would be raised. "How many of you ever expect to write a report to another doctor, a hospital, or an insurance company?" Now more hands went up. With just a few more questions, almost all of the hands in the room had been raised and there was no need for me to sermonize. My point had been made.

Unfortunately, students, as well as a lot of physicians, believe that "medical writing" pertains only to journals or books—the scientific article. There's a lot more to the field than that, as important as it is. And it will be covered in this book.

Why teach students?

First and foremost, all physicians must write. All physicians will write to other doctors, to lawyers, to government agencies, and to insurance companies, even though they may not realize it when they are students. Sometimes they will write to patients. Sometimes they will have to reply to complaints. Unfortunately, when physicians think about medical writing, they have that mental image of scientific articles. However, that is only one part of medical writing in the life of physician. Physicians (and medical students) need to learn medical writing for more reasons than that.

Unfortunately, many physicians (and medical students) are poor at medical writing. In fact, many of them are poor at any kind of writing. But since physicians are among the best "educated" professionals around (that is, they get many more years of formal education than most people), they assume that they are automatically good writers. There is good reason why they are not. The necessity for and obsession with the sciences, the dedicated concentration on these fields and the additional time needed to devote to so many other related subjects can easily keep the students from acquiring the skills needed to be good writers. They need this enormous amount of dedicated time just to absorb the necessary information and get through school.

Another assumption that interferes is that students come to medical school with intensive preparation. We believe they know all about mathematics, all about writing, all about science—but they are really just beginners in all of them.

Because doctors are assumed to be educated, it is in their best interest to be able to present to the public the appearance of being good writers, in addition to the real need in life to be able to write well.

As in everything else, the earlier we start any training, the better our success will be. It is just as true, therefore, that the earlier physicians (or medical students) begin to learn good writing the better they will eventually be.

Objectives

The objectives of this book are the same ones we might set up for a course in medical writing:

1. To familiarize, or remind, readers about the mechanics of writing medical articles and other kinds of writing

2. To suggest some specific helps in several known problem areas

3. To answer questions and to try to clear up any pre-existing difficulties

4. To raise the consciousness of the reader about medical writing. No one course or one book can teach anyone to write well. There is only one way to learn: write, write and rewrite. Use help wherever possible, either in the form of textbooks or reference books or, if available, some sort of personal help.

Part I

Scientific Medical Articles

Chapter One

What Will I Write About?

One of the most frequent questions I am asked whenever I discuss medical writing -- especially with doctors -- is, "What in the world will I write about? I'm not a research person." For some reason, the mental set of most doctors is that they think only of research when they think about medical writing. Nothing could be further from the truth.

Let's examine some of the possibilities for medical articles for physicians:

Research.

Of course, this is one of the major areas of publishing because, good or bad, most research projects wind up with some kind of scientific report. The problem in getting physicians to do medical writing is never with the research physicians because it is part of their training and part of their protocols. Research done by physicians and medical scientists is usually either in the basic sciences or in clinical research. If you decide to measure or evaluate a certain project in medicine – maybe growth of a streptococcus under certain conditions or the effect of a new drug in a particular illness -- the research paper is assumed to be part of the goal. These physicians and scientists do not need any prodding to decide what they should write about.

Clinical Practice.

To me, the larger and more important area for medical writing for physicians is the area of what I call Clinical Practice. And this offers the greatest opportunities for the majority of physicians. These would be medical reports written by doctors who are actually seeing patients and who find in their practice interesting situations that are worth sharing with their colleagues.

Two particular types of medical writing fall into this category: Case Reports and research of clinical practice:

Case Report

This basically is writing a medical report when an interesting or unusual diagnosis, finding, reaction or treatment occurs, but it must be something that is substantiated. It also offers the writer the opportunity of gaining extensive knowledge in a particular area by preparing the Case Report. Writing a case report is very rewarding and valuable enough that some graduate medical education programs require their trainees to do this exercise under supervision.

Usually, the Case Report does not arise from a planned project. Almost always, cases are reported because of unexpected or different findings, or an unusual aspect of an illness.

Example. One day I was examining a young teenager for an upper respiratory infection. As part of my usual complete examination, I was palpating her extremities and stopped short when I reached her patella. She had no kneecap (I had never heard of such a situation, obviously some knowledge I was missing). She had no kneecaps. My face must have shown my concern because her mother immediately asked "Is there something wrong?" I hesitated because I was not sure of myself and I gave her the vague answer, "I am having difficulty finding her kneecap." The mother broke out in a knowing smile and she said, "That's okay, almost everybody in our family has the same problem." As I learned later (in the confines of my library), this was Nail-Patella Syndrome. After doing the literature search, I came to the conclusion that this syndrome was rare enough to consider reporting it in the literature, even though some cases had already been reported.

Armed with her information that other members of the family had this same affliction and my literature findings that indicated this was an hereditary condition, I decided that it would be a good opportunity to do a family-tree study. I assigned a student who was on rotation in pediatrics with me to visit the child's home. The mother gathered her entire clan and the student took histories from the family, tracing which relatives were involved and to what extent. Some of these cases had already been reported, but my young patient and two others had not. This was published as "Nail-Patella Syndrome: A Report of Three Cases." This is an example of keeping alert even during the routine of regular practice to find conditions worth reporting. And it added to my knowledge.

A case report is usually the first of its kind—special symptoms not previously reported, an unusual laboratory finding, a diagnosis not previously reported, or a new or different adverse reaction to a medication or a therapy. However, it is perfectly acceptable to report the second case of its kind or a third. In some instances, there may be reason to report cases even after a number have been written up; it depends on the situation.

Research of Clinical Practice

This is best defined as a research project based on a special problem—small or large—that arises in a physician's practice, or in the doctor's fields of special interest. It will not be a major project—a cure for cancer—or a dollar-intensive program. It is usually a small project, not expensive to run, which the doctor or his office staff can do in a short time span.

Example. It might be a different approach to a special interest of the physician. While practicing pediatrics, I had a special interest in child guidance, in child psychology and the behavior problems of children. Based on that, there were several instances in which I was able to create an article based on something I did or noticed in that area of practice, something that I thought was important or of interest to other physicians.

Example. Through a series of events early in my practice, I found that weak, sweet tea was a great treatment for vomiting or diarrhea or both, without using medications. When I became satisfied that this was a reasonable therapeutic tool, I was able to produce all or part of several articles based on this special approach.

Example. Early in my internship, and with an already established interest in pediatrics, I found that I had some difficulty in interpreting blood counts in newborns. I could not follow the fluctuation of lymphocytic elements and neutrophilic elements of the blood. Going to the literature, I found that the "normals" varied from day to day in the newborn, and then week-to-week and then year-to- year up to 12 years of age—what a headache to remember unless you work with them on a daily basis. After much thought (and a little research), I devised a scheme that produced a mathematical ratio which instantaneously told the doctor whether the lymphocyte/ neutrophile ratio was normal for a particular child's age. Result: my first published scientific article "An Index for Children's Blood Counts."

Example. In a teaching conference with medical students, the question of preoperative laboratory studies in children came up for discussion. At that time, every child admitted to the hospital had a urine analysis done routinely. In our discussions, both the students and I wondered how many of those children had abnormal urinalyses and how many were followed up and found to have some renal involvement. Again, I assigned a medical student who was training with me in pediatrics to survey all of the surgical admissions in one hospital for the previous 12 months. Surprisingly, he found a large number of abnormal routine admission urinalyses and in not one single instance was a follow-up urinalysis done, even though most of the children underwent surgery anyhow. This report was never published, even though it was interesting, because we felt that for it to be a fair report, it would require intensive research into each case regarding the type of surgery, the surgeon involved, the interpretation of the attending physician/surgeon and other contributing factors. Suffice it to say that in this one hospital, at least for the children surveyed, no one paid any attention to abnormal findings on admission urinalyses.

Example. Sometimes an article may be written to call attention to a little problem which you may observe but you have not seen in the literature. Shortly after the phenothiazines were marketed as a treatment for vomiting and were being used widely in children, we made an anecdotal observation of a sudden increase of children admitted to our hospital with extra-pyramidal or Parkinson's-like syndrome. The warning about this side effect was in the original literature and in the package insert distributed by the pharmaceutical manufacturer, but with the increasing use of this drug, this syndrome also became widespread. We discussed this with the editor of a prominent pediatrics journal who noted that he had not seen any reports in the pediatric literature about this. He requested that we prepare an article reporting our observations. It appeared as "Phenothiazine Reactions in Children."

Example: In my practice, I used an infant feeding schedule that differed from most other schedules, based on some of my readings. At that time, the literature indicated great concern for Iron Deficiency Anemia occurring at 7 to 10 months of age. For prevention, routine use of an iron-supplemented milk formula was recommended. I wondered whether our different feeding schedule was the reason we did not find much of this "common" anemia in the infants in our practice. We tested 110 infants' hemoglobin levels at 7-10 months of age, and found, indeed. that our patients did not have Iron-Deficiency Anemia. Result: Another published article: "Hemoglobin Levels in the First Year of Life" – without intensive research, or grant support or any of the other trappings usually associated with doing scientific articles. But an opportunity to write something worthwhile.

Another area rife for clinical research lies in the various measurements (laboratory findings, physical measurements, developmental landmarks, for example) on children—measurements that appear to be vague or inconclusive or misunderstood or very old—or in conflict with your findings or experience. This area lends itself to research – as in our hemoglobin studies – because numbers and standards are involved, and can be compared.

All these are examples of where we found publishable material right in our own daily general pediatric practice to report on. My practice was no more esoteric or scientific or different than anyone else's – the material is there if doctors are alert to the possibilities. I apologize for citing my own cases but I did it to prove that every practicing physician can find publishable material within his or her own day-to-day practice. Whenever a physician finds an unusual case, or an unusual reaction, or unusual finding, it should be reported if it has not appeared in the literature before.

Even if these are minimal reports, it is worthy of adding your findings. It is almost as though the doctor, in reporting, is saying, "Here is a case that I had. Have any of my colleagues seen anything like this? Perhaps if they have, we may be on to something which will help many patients."

Literature Review

This is the type of medical writing that a number of physicians would like to do (or at least they talk about it), rarely do, and are not usually qualified to do. Reviews are generally comprehensive, mostly non-judgmental, balanced summaries of reports on a particular subject. It may be exhaustive or limited to a focused portion of the field. Many doctors have said, "Gee, I'd like to do an article on sinusitis in children: I see a lot of cases." Or "I'd like to write on abdominal pain in adolescents." The problems are: first, such a doctor does not focus down clearly on what he would like to do, and second, literature reviews are usually requested by editors from among top authorities in a particular field, and not usually accepted from unknowns. This is because it is expected that the reviewer be capable of weighing published facts and varying opinions.on the subject.

Actually, this is a more daunting task than writing other kinds of medical articles. The literature review portion must be an almost complete review of the subject, with almost every available reference. In most instances, a publication requires a reviewer to reach conclusions, interpret (and confirm or modify) what others are writing or add pertinent information.

This is not the place a novice should try to start medical writing.

Example. Our medical students and residents were experiencing some difficulty in interpreting the time at which various reflexes in the newborn appeared and when they disappeared. In researching the subject for answers, I was able to construct an understandable chart, and I created a literature review (that is, I did not do direct research nor add anything to the literature already out there). We just found a way to make it more understandable to trainees. We published it as "Reflexes in the Newborn."

Chapter Two

Formats for Articles

The Case Report

The Case Report is an objective presentation of a single case (sometimes multiple cases), featuring a specific finding, a different approach, or an unusual history.

The format of a Case Report is, like all other publishable medical articles, dependent on the journal to which it is being submitted. While there is a wider variance in other articles, most journals adhere to a relatively standard format in case reports. Most are based on the following outline:

> *Introduction* – a brief opening statement which tells why you chose to report this case.

> *The Case History* – the story of the particular case you are reporting, sufficient in detail for understanding but not overburdened with non-essential   information. No jargon should be

used, even though this is the place novices are most likely to use it.   (See Jargon, Chapter 6)

Discussion – in this section, the author compares the findings of the sentinel case wiith those in the literature (an expansion of why he/she chose this case to report), and why it is important. This is the "meat" of the article.

Summary – sometimes included, sometimes not. Include it only if it fits the style of the publication or is important to the point of the article.

Conclusions – it is presumptuous to try to draw conclusions from one case, or even from two or three. You are usually allowed to postulate some ideas but without being dogmatic. You may draw conclusions if you are reporting tens of cases, but even then you should be careful not to make any global assumptions -- or maybe make them tentatively.

References – should be included only if needed to justify important parts of the paper; otherwise, use no general references.

Clinical/Scientific Articles

These are the articles that make up the bulk of published medical literature. Whether the articles are written in formal style or in the newer informal form, certain parameters must be met.

First, every writer—new or old—should determine his or her objective in writing any paper. What do I want to say? What point am I trying to make? What is the relationship to present acceptable knowledge? Once an objective is chosen, keep the goal always in mind; it will force you to keep dedicated to completing the objective.

Write a brief synopsis. This is for your own use: tell yourself what you plan to say and why. Actually, it matters not whether you are an experienced author or just trying to write your first article, use of the synopsis will depend on your personality. To some writers, a synopsis will seem wasteful and non-productive, to others, valuable and pertinent -- again depending on your personality. It's up to you.

The title is very important and must be chosen wisely. In some instances, the choice of title may be delayed until after the article is written (and sometimes may be changed several times) and other times it is chosen before any words are put on paper. Or, sometimes changed by an editor after the article is accepted. This is satisfactory as long as the author follows his or her objectives. At times, the title may be assigned in advance by an editor; this situation really provides a guideline for the writer, an indication of what the editor wants in the article. In most cases, an editor will be cooperative and allow you to change what he or she has suggested, as long as it is reasonable.

Example – I once decided to do an article for a consumer magazine on the use of punishment in the rearing of children. Well up front, I chose the title "Making the Punishment Fit the Crime," at once a familiar line (Gilbert and Sullivan), a catchy one and a broad enough one to let me write what I wanted on the subject. I had a reasonable initial concept about the content and the title gave me flexibility in addition. A perfect marriage. And the editor was pleased!

Example – I repeat that the title is vital. I titled my first book "Some Uncommon Views on Some Common Problems in Pediatrics" because that was exactly what the subject material was. After accepting the manuscript, the publisher strongly recommended a change. He pointed out that books are indexed (including Index Medicus) by the first word in the title, or the first few words; that would determine the listing of the work. He made me understand that having it indexed under "Some Uncommon Views" would lead few people to read it. He suggested "Pediatrics: Some Uncommon Views on Some Common Problems." He was right!

Decide what publication you would want to submit it to—that will determine the format you use. It's important to follow the format prescribed by the particular publication. It's insulting to the journal, and to the editor, to ignore their style suggestions and use your own format. It can make them approach your article with a less-than-open mind. And if the article is good enough, the style will have to be changed anyway to fit the rest of the articles in the publication.

How do you know what style to use? Almost every publication has a page or more devoted to "Instructions to Authors" – a helpful compendium of the journal's style requirements -- and if they do not, look over the articles in a previous issue of the publication. If your article is rejected by the first publication and you have to submit it to another one, yes, you may have to do some rewriting to meet the style of the second (or third) publication; many authors before you have done this for years.

Before starting your writing, organize your data and construct rough drawings of your tables and figures, if you are using them. After all, much of what you say will be built upon those supportive graphics and numbers, so they should be clear to you. If your article does not depend on your data, graphs and tables, their information is probably not pertinent and should be eliminated.

If your article is to be an accurate and learned one, and get published, you will need to do some library work (see Chapter Four). Before any writing takes place, you should make at least a preliminary literature search, supplementing it later if necessary. Most editors will refuse an article not based on attributable facts or reliable literature sources; therefore, make this an important part of your preparation.

Whatever plan you have for the article, think about the contents of each section and actually outline it on paper. It should be brief and orderly, and most important of all, understandable to you. This will not be an iron clad restraint, because most authors find that as they write, some ideas change, and therefore you may want to change the outline, either its order or its emphasis. But it will give you a road map and keep you from straying too far off the path and wasting your precious time.

Now you should be ready to start writing. Where is that start? Probably one good piece of advice is to sit down, and write the first draft from beginning to end—without stopping to make corrections or do any editing. You should do this as fast as possible, before your thoughts dry up. You are capable of thinking probably ten times as fast as you can handwrite and maybe five times as fast as you type (or compute). Your initial rush of ideas may disappear or become confused or convoluted with any delay in writing. Let your ideas flow as freely as possible, and if, in the middle of a sentence you go blank, leave it alone and go on to the next thought. You will be surprised at how much of your original thinking and planning you can recoup with this method.

Another excellent method is to dictate rather than write. By recording, you get your thoughts down almost as fast as you think of them, and they are preserved for transcription. But again, do not go back and edit or change while dictating because it may interfere with your continuity of thought. Talk freely and as fast as possible. The time for editing will come---after your paper is transcribed. You can make all the changes and corrections you want once the first draft is on paper or on the second or third draft. Many authors find this method most helpful.

Example. My first book "Pediatrics: Some Uncommon Views on Some Common Problems" was totally dictated with a hand-held micro-cassette recorder, then typed, then edited (several times). I was completely satisfied with the process, with the speed and with the efficiency. My only dissatisfaction was that I dictated all of it while driving to and from the hospital every day — producing many distractions to me and my driving and creating potential dangers for those driving near me. (I do not advise anyone to emulate me in this!)

Technology has brought us another advance: voice-recognition computer software. With this, you can dictate to your computer while watching it come up onto the screen. You can edit whenever it is possible for you to do so --after certain time intervals, or after you have dictated a section or two. Or you can produce the entire document, print it and then do your editing. It saves an inordinate amount of time, works well and helps preserve the continuity of your thinking process.

Example. Portions of this book were done by computer-dictation and I am very satisfied, even though I am basically a computer-phobe.

Almost everybody needs to do a first draft; there are very few exceptions. Newspaper reporters, because of deadlines, are often forced to do a final draft at the first typing—often sending a page at a time to an editor or typesetter. Most of these news stories are excellent, although there are many times that reporters, in afterthoughts, wish they had the opportunity to make some changes and improvements.

In the medical field, I knew at least one outstanding exception to the multiple draft method. The late Morris Fishbein, MD, editor of the Journal of the American Medical Association for many years, and an icon and pacesetter in medical writing, used to dictate several articles each morning, give the tapes to his secretaries and never look at the manuscripts again. His writing was phenomenal.

The one counter-word to this advice is writer's block. In some cases of writer's block, my advice would be: start anyplace in the entire work, wherever your thoughts are at the moment. Then they will be sharp and will flow smoothly. Work from there. This gets you started, later you can return to writing in continuity.

IMRAD

IMRAD is an acronym which covers the usual and most common approach to writing scientific articles. Some journals will use modifications of this, but most observe these basics. IMRAD stands for Introduction, Methods and Materials, Results And Discussion.

Introduction. This is a short beginning statement which states the general field of the article so that the reader knows what is coming, if the title does not give it away. In this section, you tell the reader what you are going to do and why you are going to do it. In some instances, you may even state your assumptions or conclusions.

Methods and Materials. This essentially tells what you did and how. You explain how you conducted the research, what materials (or people) you used and what other methods were employed. The writer must decide, in advance of writing this section, who the audience will be and then peg the material to them. For example, if you are writing for trained investigators, e.g. Journal of Clinical Laboratory Investigation, this section will have to be very technical to be on the level of the reader. On the other hand, if the material is for a publication like Clinical Pediatrics, it will be much less detailed but heavy in clinical aspects.

Results. This is the section in which you present your data and the conclusions you have drawn. If there are tables, or diagrams, or figures, here is where they go. However, be sure not to repeat in writing what is obvious from the graphic data, except for over-riding findings and your conclusions from them.

Discussion. Explain the high points to the readers. Tell them what you found and why you think you found them – but not in gruesome detail. Discuss the theoretical aspects, and, where there is controversy, give both sides. Speculation is allowed but it must be reasonable, founded in your observations and subject to further testing.

Chapter Three

Where Shall I Submit It?

Ask any novice in the medical writing field where he or she is going to submit an article, or where he or she would like to submit a contemplated article, and the likely answer would be the New England Journal of Medicine or the Journal of the American Medical Association or some equally prestigious publication. When you do not know, little thought is given to where would be the *most* reasonable placement, or where it is most likely to be accepted.

Submission of an article to a highly prestigious journal is ambitious and commendable. But for many articles and for most first-time authors, it may be over-reaching. How, then, do you decide?

First, consider the kind of article. Do not submit a case history to a journal which does not use case histories—check first, read an issue of that journal. It's surprising how often this investigation is not done first, even before writing the article. Obviously, a case report of a 50-year old man would not go to a pediatrics journal, and a study of pneumonia would most likely not be submitted to a surgical journal. These parameters are fairly apparent.

Think about the scope of the article. The more universal the application, the more reason there is to consider a broad-interest publication, like NEJM or JAMA. Ah, but they also take more focused articles, usually with an eye to potential readers. A dilemma for the writer.

Sometimes politics, or special interest of the writer, plays a role. Often an author may prefer to hope for an acceptance from a journal in his specialty field rather than a more widely-read publication. Or a member may decide to bolster his or her state's journal instead of looking around for a broader readership.

Regardless, you should think carefully, and even before writing, where you would most like to have it published. Weigh all the aspects – field, specialty, scope. Remember that most journals are overloaded with submissions, so make a priority list of your preferences.

Consider your profession. For example, I would consider it foolhardy for a chiropractor, whatever his article, to submit it to a nationally famous MD publication. The likelihood of acceptance is slim.

There are two types of publications to decide between. The controlled-circulation journal ("throw-away" journal, i.e., distributed free) and paid-subscription journals obtained either by fee or as part of a membership. It has been said by some wags that the subscription journals are those the doctor keeps on his open shelf but rarely reads, and the throw-aways are those he reads but rarely saves. Joking aside, both are important and have their followings; you have to consider which you want. The controlled-circulation journal is generally less formal and therefore easier to read. It gives the writer very wide exposure but does not get listed in Index Medicus or other lists (thus persons researching the literature will not be able to locate it or identify it). They rarely use peer review. The subscription journal may be read by a narrower audience and will be much more formal in style. It is prestigious and is listed in Index Medicus. Most of these journals use peer review.

Therefore, look at the journal you have selected. Look in it for "Instructions for Authors." If there's compatibility, go ahead! But be prepared for possible rejection, or at least re-writing at the direction of the editor. Have your next choice at hand.

In writing medical articles, this may be one of the most important decisions you make!

Chapter Four

Role and Use of Library

by

Arthur A. Wachsler, PhD
Reference Librarian
Health Professions Division Library
Nova Southeastern University
and
Arnold Melnick, DO

Sooner or later – probably sooner –- anyone who does medical writing will have the need for a library. Why a person goes to the library varies with the writer—how long he/she has been writing, what the paper is about, how much need there is for specific references.

Regardless of topic or experience, whenever there is something you do not understand or need help with, **consult the Reference Librarian.** This library icon's total job (almost) is to help you find references you need. I cannot repeat that often enough.

For some articles, a writer may only need to check a definition, or a drug, or a procedure. Sometimes, the entire paper (or most of it) will require intensive literary research and use of multiple references. Review papers are almost all reference supported, as are classroom term papers.

So, too, the amount of instruction needed by a beginning writer will also vary greatly—depending on his/her library exposure. And also how sophisticated one is in modern library techniques. Thus, this work will not attempt to include a total comprehensive, all-inclusive walk through the library. What we will try to do is integrate library use with the writer's background.

Library facilities everywhere have undergone miraculous changes in this age of electronics. So jump aboard the bus at whatever your stop is.

Print searches

Those who learned library use early on will remember the relative simplicity of literature searches. Go to the Cumulative Medical Index, produced monthly by the National Library of Medicine in Bethesda. Check the topics related to your search. Then, either go to the bound-periodicals stacks and find your volume, or fill out a library request for those that are elsewhere in the building. With this material spread out before you on a library table, you could collate and select the information you so desperately needed — or go back and find more sources.

That pursuit of print references is still pure and available, but modernization through electronics has expanded the horizons, multiplied the available sources, organized more fully the existing information, and, although it may require some training, made it all more readily obtainable. And some of it you can do from your home or office—no need in many instances to go physically to the library. Because of the volume of electronic resources available, sometimes the process can become onerous – or confusing.

The Electronic Age

Today almost all medical libraries can offer electronic approaches to subject searches. However, you must develop computer skills and know how to apply them. Analogous to writing with pen and pencil or two-fingering an old typewriter, if you want the benefits of the modern age, you must learn details of the computer.

There have been developed a great number of sources of material collated under specific topics or areas of medicine – called *databases*. Then there are *search engines* which help the reader find the appropriate databases. Available are such helps as lists of print materials, reference books, dictionaries and encyclopedias, Internet links, drug and disease information, online publications and journals, and other resources There are also general guides of great import, such as BUBL LINK, Med Web and the like.

Probably the best source of all is The National Library of Medicine, which collated under Medline a compilation of over 10 million records from 4,800 journals, dating from 1966 to the present. Recently, the NLM supplemented Medline, adding records that extend the date back to 1950.

In addition, many of the major medical publications offer their issues online, including JAMA, New England Journal of Medicine, Annals of Internal Medicine and many others. One can find full texts of many textbooks, including such noted ones as Harrison's "Principles of Internal Medicine."

But where to start?

I would repeat: If you need help at any point, **consult the Reference Librarian at your library.** Or, if you are not familiar with electronic searching, consult the librarian at the very start.

Almost all Reference Librarians have created, for their specific libraries, instruction pamphlets or help sheets or instruction manuals to aid those seeking library information. Some are so detailed that they are step-by-step or "take you by the hand" guides including use of the computer and the reference searches. The Reference Librarian at your library will be happy to provide one of these and will take the time to go over it with you—or there may be classes or instructional periods available.

Among the best of these are the guides from the University of California, University of Colorado and Johns Hopkins University –remembering that each of these applies mainly to its respective university library. Your librarian will offer one appropriate for that library.

Keep in mind an important point in using these references: Through your library (university or other), most of these extensive references, including specific articles from specific journals are available at no cost. Should you feel that you want to do your work from your home computer, you must have access to your university library, or there may be charges for some of the references or materials. Again, your Reference Librarian can help you with this.

A recent development in aiding researchers is the Pathfinder or Subject Guide series These outline, by medical subject, how to go about obtaining information or accessing reference materials. Again, most of these are *specific* to a *specific* library, but in many cases include links to available sites to everyone on the Internet.

Database Safeguards

Within databases there exist safeguards to prevent using sources that are questionable. Many quality databases include "limiters." These allow the user to check off various desired categories. For example, to make sure of the quality of the article, the researcher can choose to filter the results of the search through what is known as "peer reviewed" resources. Only those articles are retrieved, then, that come from journals with high standards of research, thus eliminating substandard materials from the results.

Another filter often found in many databases is "EBM" or "Evidence-Based-Medicine." The researcher can be sure that the material retrieved is of the highest quality if it comes from the Cochrane group of databases. Only the very best articles are part of a Cochrane report, for they have been evaluated by the best authorities in Medicine. To look at a Cochrane report is to marvel at the thoroughness of the researcher.

Some individual medical libraries are transferring database presentations to electronic interactive programs that not only cover searching databases, picking on-line resources and linking to full-text articles, but also testing a student's progress toward becoming a productive and efficient user of the library's electronic resources

A little caution

An important difference exists between print references (or the electronic transcriptions of print materials) and purely electronic reports. And therein lies the need for a writer's alertness.

Print references are a permanent record, something that no one can change or modify except by creating a new print record. On the other hand, electronic references can be nebulous. For example, someone can either mistakenly or deliberately or stupidly put incorrect information on a website -- whether it be facts, background or conclusions. If it is wrong, it stays there until the error is discovered, at which point the correction can be made. And that can happen seconds after the original or weeks, months or years after. The reader may never know or realize it has been changed. The research is then left akimbo, quoting a source that no longer exists; no one can verify it and the writer may even be accused of falsifying a reference.

Nor is this problem mitigated by quoting a reference as "accessed May 1, 2005." This notation can easily be false, and does not really establish legitimacy of a reference.

A reference may be a "blind" one, having no backing in print—or in actuality. Without known background, the source may be questionable. In some instances, the "reference" may be a commercial one, with its in-built bias, or suspicion of bias..

Another detriment is that anyone -- knowledgeable or not, reliable or not, authoritative or not—can post anything he or she wants, for whatever reason, on an Internet site.

Remember always that for a reference to be acceptable, it must be able to be checked, to be challenged and, if necessary, changed.

So what is a writer to do—especially a novice? Here are some guidelines:

1. First and foremost, depend primarily on major, universally-recognized databases, such as Medline or some of its equally-respected databases. Although these, too, can be changed without notice, the likelihood of that happening is slim -- and you can pretty much depend on the reliability of government agencies, university sources and material abstracted from published books.

2. Carefully evaluate any *other* source by determining who runs the site, who pays for it and what its purpose is.

3. If necessary, check the *original* source yourself. (A good suggestion, in any case.)

4. If an Internet source seems to contradict a consensus, check it again carefully and then point it out.

5. If an Internet source is, or appears to be, a commercial one, point that out, too.

6. Remember that "personal communication" references are suspect unless the name is a well-known one and backed by status in the field.

Legitimate and recognized electronic sites are a boon to readers and writers, but care must be taken to eliminate sources that may seem, or become, questionable.

The medical library—particularly its reference section and today its electronic facility – is an indispensable tool for medical writers, whether students, novice writers or experienced authors. Just as a health professional is not expected to treat his/her own illnesses, so the writer must call frequently on that person who can help most with finding references and materials. Final word: **Consult the Reference Librarian**—sooner rather than later.

Chapter Five

The Informal Style

Within the past decade or so, a new trend has appeared in the field of medical writing. It is, more or less, informal writing. At one time, medical journals adhered to a strict format and style: formal, rigid and impersonal. Anything less would be rejected. However, in the mid-1900s, some writing authorities recognized the need for more flexibility although it took years to find its way into many publications.

Very early on, arcane language and medicalese dominated published medical articles. Many were not readable or understandable. Years ago, a subsequently world-famous physician submitted his first article to a very prestigious journal. It was immediately returned, with the following "nasty" notation: "Do you realize that any layman could understand this article?" Thank goodness, things have changed. And that physician delighted, for years, in repeating that anecdote.

Many early converts recognized that it was better to say, "I believe…" rather than the circumlocution,

"It is the opinion of the author..." a phrase that was not unusual in bygone days. Recent developments have led some recognized journals to allow more freedom –and therefore more understanding—into their publications.

Informal writing is personal and easier to comprehend, yet it must preserve the accurate and scientific. It is made up of three chief components:

1.   The use of the personal pronoun. "I", "we" and "us" are found more often today in scientific writing. It gives a composition more impact and is much more expressive and accurate than the use of third party references.

2.   It allows an author to express his opinion, without being a slave to formalism and statistics. Obviously a writer cannot make counter-assumptions in face of statistical proof, but he need not pander to each statistical item. The new style creates difficulty because some editors will not believe anything without statistical proof. The writer may not be allowed to use inferential reasoning or postulations from less-than-convincing numbers, something that has more leeway in informal style.

3.   It allows for differences in individual authors' styles, rather than a rigid formula-style, the so-called "little houses on a hillside." It is more individualistic, and therefore makes for better reading.

This does not mean a laissez-faire editorial policy of "Do what you want whenever you want." It is merely a more liberal, less restrictive, and probably more interesting and relaxed style.

I am including two extreme quotations illustrating this. They are radical, and certainly colorful. They were submitted to a journal I edited but I would not go as far as publishing them because they were too outlandish. But they were readable. They were interesting. And they were undeniably clear. Plus they are illustrative of the genre I refer to.

First, from a gynecologist:

"It was once stated by a noted gynecologist that if the ovaries occupied the same anatomic relations as the testicles, there would be a helluva lot less surgery."

Next, from a proctologist:

> "The preoccupation throughout the centuries with the vaginal introitus has made a second-rate citizen of the anal outlet, slightly south of its border. Modern mores, with its emphasis on instant sex, had tended to blunt the problem further, but the puckered neighbor has not changed its geography one iota. In fact, its unpredictable rumbling protest may be a social catastrophe, despite elastic, plastic and perfume."

What would be publishable, in this vein?

Try this from a gynecologist:

"Personally, if I see a patient with a small fibroid and she is desirous of taking the "pill", I select an agent with the lowest content of estrogen and progestin having the highest anti-estrogenic potency."

Is that precise and exact? There is no question of what that gynecologist would do for the patient.

Yes, the informal can be scientific. It can be precise and exact. It can be more colorful. And it can be clear.

Chapter Six

Pitfalls in Exposition

Exposition is the art of writing to explain a subject. To study it thoroughly requires understanding of thousands of rules and protocols. They are not within the province of this book. I will not attempt to be global and comprehensive. This is not a grammar book. I have chosen areas of writing that I think are quite important and which are frequently ignored by health students or beginning medical writers. And there are parts of this serious discussion that can be fun.

How to Write (Review of Exposition)

It is important that those aspiring to be medical writers learn some of the important principles of good writing, practice them and learn some of the common problems evidenced by other writers still learning the trade.

Note the title of this section. It carries two implications, both mean the same. "Review of

Exposition" is correct. It is formal and depends on bigger words. "How to Write" says it more clearly, more understandably and uses simpler words. This illustrates the theme of this section.

First, let me make a reference to what I have called for more than 25 years Melnick's Theory[1]. It is meant to give succinctly a compressed philosophy and approach that will help beginners: Write Like You Talk (1). It was interesting to find recently "If You Can Talk, You Can Write,"[2] a splendid book published in 1993 by writing guru Joel Saltznan. It got great reviews and emphasizes the same point I am making, carrying it to even greater detail.

Most of us communicate better when talking than when writing. We can explain a simple item while speaking and the listener will understand immediately. When we write—and doctors are especially guilty of this—we suddenly transform that simple speech into complicated multi-syllabic writing. The dictum essentially says that, and tells the learner to keep it simple.

Write Like You Talk means talk to your reader, tell him what you want to say. <u>Communication is the name of the game.</u>

How do you go about doing that?

Forget the editorial "we"

Forget the impersonal pronoun

Forget the third person approach

Forget the circumlocution

Forget the passive verbs

We don't talk like that. We don't usually use those constructions. Why write like that?

Beginner's guidelines

Rules sometimes get boring, but I want to present several short ones that will go a long way toward good writing, and they are easy to remember.

Use shorter words. If faced with the decision between a short word or a long word, almost always choose the short one. A patient <u>has</u> chest pain; he doesn't <u>possess</u> it. A surgeon reaches the <u>end</u> of the operation; he doesn't reach the <u>termination.</u>

Use shorter sentences. Long sentences are more difficult to read -- and to understand. Break your thoughts into smaller sections. Make separate sentences out of them. They will carry more power.

Use familiar words. Avoid unfamiliar or far-fetched ones. One physician wrote on a patient's chart, "The patient experienced singultus." No. "The patient had hiccups."

Avoid the passive voice (using a form of the verb to be). Don't say, "Three tumors were found," say "We found three tumors." Instead of "It was observed by the author," write, "I observed" (or "We observed" if multiple authors). How much clearer and more direct. Embryonic authors often shy away from the personal pronoun; it is now acceptable in scientific writing. (See The Informal Style, Chapter 5.)

Use strong nouns and verbs. Use them instead of adjectives and adverbs. Not "Time passed very quickly" but "Time flew."

Use English forms instead of Latin. Say skin instead of dermis, head instead of caput. Beginning writers have a tendency to use many Latin forms, not out of pomposity but because they believe it is more scientific. Again, this ties in with the rule of Keep It Simple. Some writers often make this same error with non-scientific material:

> "Per" – Use "Five milligrams a vial" not "Five milligrams per vial"

> "Via" – Use "I gave him Lasix by injection" not "I gave him Lasix via injection"

Say it in English, if possible.

However, there are some Latin expressions (mainly abbreviations) that still serve a good purpose. Examples are:

> i.e. – id est ("that is," followed by a further explanation of the material).

> e.g. – exempli gratia ("for example" followed by examples)

And be sure to use commas after each of those. These are among the most frequently used. However, it must be emphasized that a common mistake is to use these interchangeably. They are not the same; you must learn where to use each. Often writers confuse these two.

Construct sentences carefully

One of the most frequently recurring errors – and often committed by established authors as much as by inexperienced writers—is the lack of agreement between the subject of the sentence and a following pronoun, e.g., (Aha! here e.g. is used correctly) "The patient told the doctor their symptoms." Patient is singular and therefore it should be "his" or "her" symptoms.

Be sure your thoughts are expressed clearly. Clarity is the keynote of all good writing. Unclear wording usually means unclear thinking. Two things result. First, the sentence is difficult for the reader to understand and to interpret. Second, sometimes humorous (or embarrassing) ideas result:

"A medical dilating instrument, the bougie, is originally a French word."

> (Unfortunately, "a medical dilating instrument" is not a French word, but *bougie* is originally a French word.)

"Television requires little mental activity, and in my opinion this is what we need." ("Mental activity" is what we need; the indefinite article "this" in the sentence refers to "Television requires little mental activity.")

> "The children had scattered small pieces of bread among the ducks which they had been eating all afternoon." (No, not eating the ducks, but eating small pieces of bread all afternoon.)

In thinking about clarity, consider one of the glaring mistakes of beginning writers and a few experienced

ones. It is called officially "The dangling participle."
It represents first the incorrect use of an "-ing" word,
and technically, it represents lack of agreement between
the participle and the subject following it (noun or
pronoun).

> Look at this sentence: "Looking through the
> microscope, the cells appeared red." Actually,
> "cells" is the subject of the sentence, but the
> cells are not "Looking through the microscope,"
> as the sentence clearly says. Correcting it: "Seen
> through the microscope, the cells appeared
> red."

> Now, try this one: " After closing the incision,
> the patient was placed in the recovery room"
> The surgeon closed the incision, not the patient,
> so a slight change will make the sentence
> correct: "After the surgeon closed the incision,
> the patient was placed in the recovery room."

Another frequent – and very frequent—over-use is
clichés. I define a cliché as an expression or description
which has been used so often that it is worn thin, it is
hackneyed, or worn out, so that everyone knows it and
it carries very little strength of meaning or descriptive
power. Examples: "Aggressive surgical attack," " out
of the mouths of babes"(see below), and "as hard as
nails." I'm sure every reader can think of tens more
clichés—you might even find a few in my writing in this
book – after all, they are not as *scarce as hen's teeth.*
Risky as it may seem, I shall try to pick—from
among the thousands—some of the common clichés,
just so you will recognize one each and every time

you go *back to the drawing board*. Isolated from sentences, they are better recognized as clichés, and often humorous:

> A change of scene
> Agree to disagree
> Allow nature to take its course
> Beat a dead horse
> Breathe her last breath
> By and large
> Caring physicians
> Cool as a cucumber
> Dead of the night
> Fools rush in
> Grave concern
> It behooves
> Leave no stone unturned
> Loosened her tongue
> Moment of truth
> On the whole
> Proof of the pudding
> Therapeutic dilemma
> This moment in time
> Tradition of excellence
> Wonder drug

One last thought on this subject. Every word you write should be there for its exact meaning. Exact, not almost. That is one reason why the writer's most important tool is not this book, not a grammar text, not a set of writing instructions, but a dictionary. I have, right at my desk, several dictionaries and thesauruses – which I use regularly. No author should attempt to write without a dictionary or even two at his or her hand. Rare, indeed, is the writer who can complete an opus without referring to a dictionary at least a few times—and for the beginner, many more times than that. And sometimes, a meticulous writer might spend an inordinate time with the dictionary seeking a special word with the exact meaning needed. While I shall present what I hope is a helpful bibliography at the end of this book, the primary, and most important, reference for writers is a dictionary.

Out of the pens of neophytes (not *mouths of babes*)

Having taught medical writing to medical students for ten years, and having them prepare articles as assignments, I have found a number of errors being regularly repeated. These are reasonably consistent from year to year and from class to class. I have compared the students' recurring errors with those I have seen in many years of editing and they are comparable. Examples below illustrate some of the commonest pitfalls. They are not necessarily taken from students' papers but are best for illustrative purposes:

Ambiguous Sentences

> "He was treated at University Hospital since his shooting by a surgeon."

> "The malignant growth was favorably affected by x-ray."

> "The child was placed in a vaporizer."

> "The patient complained of no pain."

"A 3-month old girl presented herself because of a vaginal tumor."

"The child was discharged to be closely followed by her pediatrician."

"Patient has chest pain if he lies on his left side for over a year."

"On the first day, the elbow was better, and on the fourth day, it disappeared."

"When she was admitted, her rapid heart had stopped, and she was feeling much better."

Agreement in Number

"A patient wants to feel content with their physician"

"He spends quality time with the patient to answer their questions."

Trite

"This author believes…"

"One should consider…"

"I would like to take this opportunity…"

Punctuation

"Take, for example, our implied expectations of two individuals; one a banker, the other a doctor." (needs a colon or a comma after "individuals", not a semi-colon).

"His doctors only gave him six months to live, however, his spirits were up after his surgery, he was determined to beat the disease." (Does "however" go with the first phrase or the second one? It needs a semi-colon after "live")

Some humorous results with wrong punctuation:

"Let me call you, sweetheart"

"What's the latest, dope?"

Other frequent mistakes: missing colons and semi-colons; hyphens; and quotations within quotations

Long Sentences

One student submitted an essay with a 52-word sentence, others with 48 and 43.

Long Paragraphs

One student submitted a 400-word paragraph, others 250 words.

Apostrophes

Referring to an experience of Norman Cousins: "Cousin's" (It should be: Cousins')

"Consider the patients panic" (Needs an apostrophe between "patient" and "s" – or after the "s" depending on meaning)

"Treatment will relieve it's inflammation" (Possessive of "it" does not take an apostrophe. "It's" must only be used in the sense of "It is".)

Split infinitives (where split does not clarify)

"The physician must be able to clearly explain the disease." (Better to say "to explain the disease clearly.")

"…to not only address…" ("to address not only…")

Non-sentences (fragments)

"Thereby allowing the doctor to conduct an examination."

"Both of which need to be avoided."

"Thus creating a sense of urgency."

Spelling confusion

Affect vs. effect

Allude vs. elude

They're vs. their vs. there

Site vs. cite

Lie vs. lay

Principal vs. principle

Infer vs. imply

Spelling errors

Flehm

Decifer (Decipher)

Differance

Inexact expressions

"The doctor dilated the patient's pupil" not "The doctor dilated the patient"

A doctor will "follow a case" but will "observe the patient" (He will not "follow the patient")

Some more gaffes

Most of us, sooner or later will fall into the chasm of these writing errors. Conscious as we might be about them, they tend to slip into our writing, and our speaking, more often than we would like. Most important is to be constantly aware of them and try to stay alert.

Wordy phrases

This is saying more than is needed, instead of being concise and more precise. Compare the wordy phrases on the left with the better way to say it on the right:

It is clear that	Clearly
It is obvious that	Obviously
It must be admitted that	Admittedly

It is undoubtedly true that	Undoubtedly or Doubtless
It is now considered possible that	Possibly
At the present time	Now or Currently
Subsequent to	After

Note also that the first five also violate the rule of avoiding the passive voice.

Useless modifiers

This is an exercise in redundancy. In each instance, the writer wrote more than was necessary, and, in fact, duplicated the first description. Obviously, these are only a handful of samples; many, many other violations occur daily.

visible to the eye	completely indispensable
oval in shape	cools off
light green in color	surrounded on all sides
few in number	entirely complete
important essentials	urgent emergencies
intradermal skin tests	gastritis of the stomach

One note of importance. I have recommended earlier in this book to Write Like You Talk. Unfortunately, these redundant expressions are a common part of our ordinary speech, so if you follow my advice, you still have to check carefully to avoid these mistakes.

Picking the right word

> Dose – dosage
> Autopsied – biopsied
> Mucus – mucous

What's the plural?

> Dat…index…
> Criter…phenomen…

"Case"

Rarely do you focus on just a single word, but the overworked word "case" is one that justifies such attention. Most of the errors with "case" occur in medical writing.

First, we mention it to decry referring to patients as cases. We tend to write "This case recovered," "We gave antibiotics to this case" or "This case in Room 302." Reference to patients as cases should be eliminated. They are people, not cases.

Second, "case" meaning "occurrence" is terribly overworked, particularly since there are so many options and substitutes, to wit:

In all cases	Always
In case	If
In many cases	Often, Frequently
In some cases	Sometimes
It is often the case that	Often

How much smoother and clearer the shorter form is, and see how it eliminates the word "case."

Jargon

Jargon could be defined as a hybrid language used for special conversations between people – a sort of shorthand made up of technical terminology, maybe shortened and twisted. Each user may understand the language but it may confuse outsiders. "I gave the post-op an IV with 5 in water after she came back from the OR so don't cath her." Clear enough to the two communicants (in most instances), but totally confusing to the lay listener. And how bad it is when one of our students or colleagues tries to do medical writing this way. Some examples of jargon (among the many):

CBC	Sub-Q
Patient was diagnosed	Patient was injected
Tapped the knee	Lymphs (for cells)
Lab	Exam
Chemo - for chemotherapy	and/or
Y/o – for year old	etc.

Here's an example in a sentence, showing the wrong (funny) result: "The pelvic examination will be done later on the floor." Here's another: "Our surgeon suggested we sit tight on the abdomen, and I agree." As I stated, this jargon may be understood by another professional in medicine in brief conversation, but certainly it is not to be used in medical writing.

Also, at times, such sort-cuts can be confusing or even dangerous. MS is jargon for morphine sulfate but MS is also jargon for multiple sclerosis. It is also, at times, used to represent mitral stenosis and musculoskeletal. In a rapid-fire exchange, or in a crisis situation, there could be misunderstanding and trouble. There are many other jargon words or expressions which have more than one meaning. Some examples:

AP – anterior-posterior, auscultation and percussion, appendicitis

BP – blood pressure, benzoyl peroxide, British Pharmacopeia

CAT – computed axial tomography, Children's Apperception Test, cataract

HD – hearing distance, Hodgkin's Disease, hemodialysis

ID – intradermal, infectious disease, initial dose

TT – transtracheal, thrombin time, tetanus toxoid

Confusing? Yes and that confusion can lead to dangers for patients. For writers, it is a no-no because the readers may not understand.

Let's Laugh at Ourselves (and the things we write)

Two pearls that I have come across illustrate clearly some of the errors, emphasizing them through humor.

Many years ago, a contributor to a publication I edited sent me a list purporting to show some of the ways we as writers use devious routes of expressing ourselves, and what the real meanings are:

Term	Meaning
1. Cases drawn from our clinical experience	1. I've got two
2. Review of the literature reveals	2. Mayo's has two

3. Extensive review of the literature reveals

3. Mayo's has two and Punjab University has 63

4. The equipment was modified to our specifications

4. The instrument was dropped on the floor

5. The equipment was found satisfactory in its original design

5. The instrument was not dropped on the floor

6. The patients were lost to follow-up evaluation

6. They skipped town without paying their bill

7. Some resistance was met at an administrative level

7. It scared the hell out of the DME

8. Delay was encountered in obtaining proper equipment

8. I bought it on time

9. Most investigative work has been done in this country

9. a) I don't read German, or

b) I do read German but it isn't worth it, or

c) If those boys from Tokyo ever publish, we can all pack up and go home

10. It is felt that further investigation will be necessary before full clinical trials are warranted	10. Oh hell, back to the drawing board

In reading these and seeing some of the possibilities, you can easily recognize a certain amount of double-talk or arrogance that go into some of these statements. While we realize that most statements like this represent true and honest findings, a reader cannot decipher which ones mean a cover-up for the truth. I am indebted to that anonymous contributor (and I am still laughing).

The second list, which is really fun-grammar, was originated by a Gyles Brandeth (source unknown).

<u>Rules of the Game</u>

1. Don't use no double negatives
2. Make each pronoun agree with their antecedent
3. Join clauses good, like a conjunction should
4. About them sentence fragments
5. When dangling your participles
6. Verbs has to agree with their subjects
7. Just between you and I, case is important too
8. Don't write run-on sentences they are hard to read
9. Don't use commas, which aren't necessary
10. Try not to ever split infinitives
11. It is important to use your apostrophe's correctly

12. Proofread your writing to if any words out
13. Correct spelling is esential

References

1. Melnick, Arnold: Platitudinous Garrulities Ain't Readable. Bethesda. American Medical Writers Association, 1973.
2. Saltzman, Joel: If You Can Talk, You Can Write. New York. Warner Books, 1993.

Chapter Seven

What Happens After You Write It?

So, you've finished writing it—whether a book or a journal paper. You've gone over it, edited it, re-written it. Now you think it's ready for publication. What happens next?

That depends. It depends on whether you have been commissioned to write it, that is, requested or contracted by a publisher or journal editor to write the work. If so, the path is easy: just send the completed work to that publisher, in the form originally requested. Usually that means typed or computer-printed, on one side of the paper, in the style of the journal, with or without a cover page (as instructed). In today's market, the publisher will probably instruct you to submit a computer floppy disk in addition to the hard copy. You've already had the question of "Where to send it?" answered for you.

But if you haven't been commissioned, you have a first and important step to take, and the decision rests on whether it is a book or a journal article.

As this is an introductory book, it cannot serve as an instructional thesis on where and how to submit. For that, there are good sources, such as "The Writer's Handbook", or "The Writer's Market," or "Literary Marketplace" which are produced annually listing journal, magazine and book publishers with an indication of what each is looking for. They are not strictly for medical writing, but can be helpful. Or talk to your medical librarian. Or consult an experienced friend or colleague. Or, for a book, examine the shelves of your local major bookstore. The compendiums mentioned contain, in addition to lists of publishers, instructional articles written by experienced authors that are valuable for the novice. Most medical publishers will provide you with (and prefer) an outline of points to do a book proposal for them. Follow their recommendations.

What will you be looking for? The best possible professional fit: A book publisher who does books in the subject area of your manuscript or related areas and one who publishes for professionals or for consumers, depending on what group your book is in.

For journal manuscripts, look around for those publications that directly pertain to your subject field. Do they publish only research or also clinical material? Do they publish case histories, if yours is such? Obviously, the closer your article fits the publication, the higher the probability that it might be accepted. Remember that journals always receive many more manuscripts than they possibly can publish, so there is stiff competition. Almost every new author sets his or her sights on journals like New England Journal of Medicine, JAMA or other highly prestigious publications. That's a commendable goal, but the competition is greatest there and it seems that the best known writers get published (maybe because they have something special to say or a special way of saying it, compared to a novice). That does not mean you shouldn't try them if, after a careful study, you think they are the most appropriate fit. However, there are many other splendid journals worth trying, if they fit your subject.

When it gets to the Publisher

Let's talk about unsolicited or non-commissioned material. You've picked a journal or publisher to send your work to, and you've submitted it. Now what?

While publishers use multiple and varying staff organizations and systems for handling manuscripts, a certain few functions are usually uniform throughout the industry:

> Decision maker – a chief editor, or publisher, or manuscript editor or other authority who makes the judgment to accept or reject the manuscript by evaluating such things as content, originality, organization, competition, logic and quality of writing. This job may be titled Acquisitions Editor.

> Working editor – copy editor or manuscript editor, who corrects the manuscript in detail or suggests changes or raises questions with the author, and who will continue to work with the author until the manuscript is totally satisfactory. This person does the nitty-gritty needed to get

the manuscript into shape, including correctness and consistency.

<u>Mechanical phase</u> – includes book design, typesetting (usually by computer), art work, paper, printing and binding.

I have purposely used descriptive functions rather than common or recognizable titles, in order for the reader to understand the process better.

These are generic job functions but, depending on the publisher or editor, most publications (called refereed journals) use a peer-review system. Your article, somewhere early in the process, is submitted to 1 to 3 or more experts in the field – anonymously. Neither referees nor writer are known to the other. After careful review, these referees provide their opinion on suitability of publishing your article, sometimes with recommendations.

Referee recommendations usually fall into three groups: (1) do not publish; (2) publish as written; or (3) publish if revised (anywhere from a minor change to a complete overhaul). A referee's written responses or comments are usually included and sent to the writer -- also anonymously.

If revision or change are called for, you as the author can say, "Yes", then revise and resubmit, or you can say, "No" and submit it to another publication.

Some publishers combine the editorial functions into fewer jobs, some divide them into many different levels, but the functions remain the same. Somewhere along this procedure, the publisher or one of his editors will be in touch with the author and guide him or her through the process—different publishers will contact the writer at different phases.

Two caveats

First, I believe the biggest surprise for first-time authors is this: No matter how much rewriting you have done, no matter how many times you have gone over it, no matter how outstanding you think the writing is, there is high probability that the publishers and editors will want to make a number of changes. In addition, an editor is cognizant of a dozen or so parameters needed to produce good and accurate copy. That is not because your work is not good; they wouldn't have accepted it if that were true. We all—every author—make some mistakes—grammar, punctuation, word choice that have to be corrected. Plus every publisher has a standard style. Your manuscript must fit that.

Example. I like occasionally to use a conjunction (but, and, or) to start a sentence for emphasis—and it is grammatically correct to do so. However, some publishers have a standard style that prohibits that use of conjunctions, and you have to go along with your publisher's style. That's so the publisher's uniform style is preserved in all the company's books.

Be prepared to accept changes in your work. They will come. And most of the time, they will improve your manuscript, even though you may at first be upset by them.

Because of all these reasons, authors should expect, for the most part, to be requested to explain or rewrite or change portions. In most instances, the editor will be in constant touch, and work with the author until the manuscript is "perfected."

The second caveat is that every new author believes his or her manuscript is so good that it will be accepted by the first publication to which it is submitted. Not true. Rarely true. Scientific or professional manuscripts, like other literary works, often undergo multiple submissions before being accepted. I do not know whether anyone has ever calculated an average number of submissions, but for non-professional articles or books, tens of submissions are not unusual, occasionally hundreds, so be prepared with a list of back-up publications to submit to, you may need them.

Every writer should develop patience. Considering the process a publisher goes through to decide on a submission, there are often long delays in getting a response.

Part II

Other Medical Writing

Chapter Eight

General Comments

As I have said, too often the term Medical Writing means to doctors and students, regardless of what discipline they represent, the authoring of medical articles for publication in a journal or book.

This definition would limit Medical Writing to a small percentage of health professionals—as not that many of us write journal articles or books. Unfortunately for those who believe this definition, it is not true. Every health care professional—physician, pharmacist, dentist, optometrist, podiatrist and all others—will in his or her professional career write many times as much other professional communication as medical articles.

To some extent, this type of writing—communication, if you will -- ultimately may be more important to professionals than articles or books. It is their day-to-day existence. It may determine payment of bills, avoidance of law suits, development of interprofessional relations, transmission of important information, retention of patients and a myriad of other benefits. In all these channels, there exists the possibility of the embarrassment of having your communication downplayed because of inability to write properly.

This section is dedicated to offering some thoughts, hints and ideas about other medical writing and I hope that all the readers will benefit by this part II. More in this section than in Part I, strategies and logic and substantive aspects of writing are included. Writing is not just the mechanics of proper grammar and correct punctuation, it includes what to write and how to write it effectively.

It would seem easy to cover this topic merely by repeating everything already said in the previous section. And that would be accurate. Or, even just calling the reader's attention to Part I again. For everything said about medical articles is true of other medical writing (with a few additions).

What do you need? In just three words: Clarity, Brevity and Completeness.

Chapter Nine

Charts, Records and Reports

Cavalierly, you could say, " If my article or book is not clear enough, not brief enough or not complete enough for the reader, tough for him." But if your charts, records or reports are not clear enough, brief enough or complete enough for the reader, and some problem arises, as it often does, then it's tough for you. So there's almost a defensive need for accuracy and thoroughness in all your writings.

Of all the requirements, probably *clarity* is the most important. What you write must be clear to every person who reads it—patient, another health professional, an insurance company, a lawyer, a judge, a jury, a medical discipline committee, a governmental agency, or whoever. No ambiguity. No misunderstandings.

Some learned people have said that if the writing is not clear, then the thinking is not clear. That attitude automatically prejudices the reader against you (if you are the unclear writer), and certainly that will be of no help to your communication. I happen not to agree with that assumption. I have seen professionals who write clearly in spite of thinking that is muddled, and I have seen clear thinkers who cannot get their thoughts on paper in a clear manner – probably because they are intimidated by the process of writing.

Brevity, the second of the three important attributes, is a two-edged sword: If your writing is not brief enough (and thus probably filled with unessential or convoluted information), it will cause several unwanted effects: it will confuse the reader, it will waste the reader's time and it will anger the reader. Put that in the context of a legal confrontation, an insurance disagreement or an unhappy patient's refusal to pay, and you'll get an immediate picture. So, your writing on charts, records and reports must be long enough to be inclusive of all necessary information yet brief enough for the reader not to be unhappy with it.

In all the situations just described, the need for *completeness* becomes obvious. Since we never know which writings will eventually become problems, all of them should be complete.

Several important considerations apply to this form of writing:

Use appropriate medical terminology. Avoid jargon and convoluted medical expressions. If writing to fellow professionals, use accurate medical terms. Avoid trying to impress. If writing to patients, be sure to explain carefully in non-medical terms, but be sure your translations are accurate: peritonitis is not a "bowel problem" or a 'bellyache" but "an inflammation of the lining of the abdomen". If you are in doubt, try it on your secretary, your spouse, or your family for understanding.

Complete accuracy. If the patient has hypertension, do not record "slightly elevated blood pressure" or "quite elevated blood pressure." Be precise: "This lady had a blood pressure of 190/120." Laboratory results should be reported in specific numbers. You will probably be lucky in adversarial situations if the readers of your writing assume you are merely unable to write clearly, rather than assume you are trying to be deceitful.

Use only standard diagnoses. This is often difficult because we all use so much jargon and verbal shorthand that we may slip easily into inaccurate diagnosis. Be sure your diagnosis is standard and universally acceptable.

Include a treatment plan. Especially in complicated instances, presence of a treatment plan (or follow-up plan) on the patient's chart (office or hospital) is important. It shows clarity of thinking and gives everyone something against which to measure the progress of the patient. Avoid vagueness and double talk.

Be specific about medication. Give names and doses. Do not assume that just because you <u>always</u> prescribe 50 milligrams of Zoloft that every reader (lawyer, judge, etc.) will accept that as truth when you say so. And your notes should never say "Z Rx". Not everyone will accept your claim that the letter "Z" represents Zoloft at 50 milligrams.

Include notes on communication. For your own peace of mind, your own remembrance and your own legal safety, always indicate in writing what you told the patient or anyone who accompanies the patient. It might also help to state whether they understood or the participant replies.

Write legibly. This is a legal precaution: always assume you are writing this for a judge to read, and you do not want him to be unable to read it. In an even worse scenario: In a deposition or trial, you are asked to read your notes and *you* are uncertain of what it says. Next case.

In writing progress notes, whether on your office chart or a hospital chart, or on any other kind of record, always assume that every record may be read at some time in the future, under some unknown or adverse circumstances, by the patient, the family, an attorney, a judge, a jury or a medical discipline committee. That means you need intelligible writing and correct grammar, in order to get Clarity, Brevity and Completeness.

Reports

By my definition, a report is a communication, usually about a patient, from one health professional (or institution) to another health professional (or institution).

Everything said about charts and records, and everything said about medical writing, is as applicable to reports. The written transfer of information –case report, consultation report or recommendations— represents you and your reputation on a written and permanent basis.

With that in mind, you will want it to be accurate, but also written in at least near-perfect grammar and punctuation. Accuracy goes almost without saying, but you do not want outside readers ever to get an impression that you are not totally literate. It can decrease your image in third-party eyes.

A few specific recommendations are important for Reports:

Sign all letters. While this may seem obvious, and it is rare for a report not to contain a signature, it does happen occasionally. Whether you accidentally forgot to sign, or for some arcane reason deliberately neglected to sign, the effect is the same: it's negative. The reader will have several questions. Did he purposely not sign and why? Does he not want to take responsibility for the contents? Is he too busy or indifferent? Don't let this happen.

Use professional stationery. A report on other than professional stationery will raise eyebrows. The same questions raised in signature may occur here also. In today's market, with computers doing so much for us, there may be a tendency to depend on computer-produced letterheads. That is satisfactory if they have a uniform appearance, are consistent and have a professional look.

Apply all writing rules. Because a report is the face you give publicly to your work, you will want to utilize all parameters of good writing. Put your best face forward—and be sure everyone will understand what you write.

Proofread every letter before it goes out. It is presumptuous and arrogant to assume that your dictation is perfect and that none of your secretarial staff will ever make any mistakes in transcribing or typing. None of us is that good; everyone makes mistakes from time to time. And a mistake in a medical-type report can affect the patient's health or even life. For example, I may want to say "prednisolone" but unconsciously it comes out "prednisone," and I won't be aware of the slip of tongue. Or, my secretary hears one word and thinks it is the other. There has developed a cadre of doctors whose letters state, "Dictated but not read" with the anticipation that it prevents responsibility or potential lawsuits. Whether it does or not, there are more compelling moral reasons and medical responsibilities that this should never be done. You owe it to your patient, you owe it to your referring doctor and, more important, you owe it to yourself to proofread the final copy – so that it is accurate.

Chapter Ten

Doctors' Letters

It is always important to remember what the purpose of your letter is. Its task is to communicate, with all the nuances implied in that. It serves to transmit a message or to send information to the reader. In some instances, a secondary purpose may be to convince someone of something, to sell something or to influence someone, but these also require the same emphasis. Since many books have been produced on letter writing, here we will limit our presentation to some highlights, especially for health professionals.Students and novices in any health profession almost never realize or understand the large number of letters they will write in their professional lives. Often, many will say, "But I'm not going to do much writing when I'm in practice," because mostly, they only consider writing in relation to medical articles or books. Today, communication by letter is a very important aspect of practice and occupies much more time and effort than expected. And the exigencies of today's medical world have increased that volume.

Types of letters

Reports. As indicated before, these are mainly consultations, or summaries of patients' records, either for transfer of the patient, submission of information or as a referral.

Complaints. In the life of a health professional, there will be many times that it is necessary to write a letter of complaint: poor quality of supplies, malfunctioning equipment, improper billing, inadequate payment and many more. Some of this will be of a professional nature, such as care of a patient in the hospital, difficulty with a colleague's actions, or of a business nature such as billing or purchases.

Congratulatory. Occasions are frequent for the writing of congratulatory letters. Patients get married, residents win awards, students have babies, employees need commendation—a myriad of instances where such a letter is appropriate, and appreciated. Sure, you can send a greeting card. But how much better is it to write a personal note and to be able to make it a clear message. A little ingenuity in writing the letter—making it a little different from trite expressions so often used—will win hearts and appreciation.

References and recommendations. Similarly, there are numerous times these letters are needed: office employees, hospital workers, other professionals and friends among others. These are really sales letters. If you want that person to get the appointment or position, the better the letter the greater the chances. However, never write derogatory letters for a reference. If you don't want that person to get the appointment—and there are such occasions when you cannot turn the person down -- your letter must be even more carefully worded, because of legal implications. One physician, asked for a reference letter for a past, disliked employee, wrote, "You will be very lucky to get this lady to work for you." Good writing, either way, is a requirement.

Applications and acceptances. Frequently, health professionals (or patients) need such letters. They apply for memberships, positions, grants. They recommend applicants for admission to schools and residencies. Such letters must also fulfill the tenets of good writing.

Organizational. Most health professionals are members of at least one organization. Many of them take part in activities, serve on committees, act as officers. In every aspect of organizational life, the writing of letters is an important part. Write to your committee members. Write to invite speakers. Correspond with those speakers regarding details. Discuss appointments. Review actions of boards. It is a limitless list, and one which requires good writing skills to be successful.

Parts of a Letter

It would be a reasonable assumption that all health professions students -- with their intensive educational backgrounds — would bring with them full knowledge of what a letter is, of what parts it is composed, and how it is set up mechanically. And most of them do. However, my experience in giving letter-writing assignments to my classes in Medical Writing is that some students do require additional instruction or refreshers in this area. Since this book is a primer, I shall include this information for those who need it.

Date. Any time you forget to date a letter is the time you will be unable to remember and you will be sorry. Always put the date on everything.

Name and address. There are two reasons. The first is to be sure you have properly addressed the recipient and second so that your records are intact about whom it was sent to.

Attention line/Reference line. This line will be a quick reminder to you in looking at the letter later, and it will notify the receiver who should be getting the letter or what the subject is.

Salutation. Some modernists believe that the "Dear George" can be left out—after all, you have greeted him in the name and address. Purists would differ. I would suggest that you use the style you are most comfortable with. One place that it would be comfortable to leave it out is when addressing a letter to a company or organization when you do not know what person should get it. For example, you write to Acme Trucking Company but do not know to whom it should go. Do you say, "To Whom It May Concern"? Or "Dear Ladies/Gentlemen"? Or "Dear Ladies and Gentlemen"? Or "Dear Sir/Madam"? or what? How much easier just to say Acme Trucking Company and start your letter without a salutation.

Body. There are usually three parts to the body. The first paragraph should gain the attention of the reader and send your message—either a quick summary, or the topic or purpose of the letter, as an introduction of the subject of the letter to the reader. This would include reference to the patient's visit or noting that a consultation on Mrs. Marie Smith was done (or, in other kinds of letters, an attention-getter of some kind, such as, "Do you know you can save money on your medical expenses?").

The middle or body of the letter is one or more paragraphs detailing the substance of the message and should be written in an orderly progression.

Part three is a summary or conclusion or both (or a call to action). This last paragraph is generally a summary of what was said in the letter (or a strong statement for action, such as, "Call me at once", or as lawyers like to say, "Please be forewarned!"). In a consultation, for example, summarize your diagnosis, treatment or recommendations or all of them:

Complimentary closing.   You have a choice of many possibilities, from the formal and austere "Yours very truly" to the very informal and personal "Affectionately". The choice of appropriateness is yours. Here too, some people today feel that the complimentary closing is an anachronism and not needed -- just sign the letter. What you do is your choice.

Signature. It would be nice if health professionals could sign their names legibly, but every letter should be actually signed even though the professional's full name and title will be typed on the letter.

Some general rules

Don't assume your letter will be read. Most of us make that assumption. But stop and review what you have done with the last ten letters you have received (not advertisements). Some you read every word because the author or the subject was of interest to you. Some you probably skimmed through, because you had a pretty good idea what they were about or the details weren't important to you. Some you may even have put away or tossed because of the writer or the subject and you felt you didn't want to waste your time ("Gee, this guy is still bothering me for a contribution!" "Oh, that lady still wants her job back!") Few letters are read completely, many only partially. That should tell you something: If you want your correspondents to read your letters, learn to get the reader's attention and keep it by making the letter pertinent and interesting, being brief enough and by making the writing appealing.

Don't be trite or pompous. Your letters will become trite if you write similar messages the same way every time—that is, if you develop a form. This is a real turnoff whether or not it really is a form letter or writing laziness on your part. One great example is the doctor, and there are many, who starts every consultation letter with "I saw your interesting patient today." The first time I received such a letter from such a consultant I was flattered that he thought my patient interesting. The second time, I was also pleased. But when it came with every consultation, I knew it was bull and flattery, and it never impressed me again.

Pomposity also has no place. It is fine to be self-centered, but to write that "Your patient got to me just in time; I saved his life" is to exaggerate most of the time. And our impression of a doctor goes down if he or she exhibits this pomposity regularly. So, don't try to impress your reader, don't be over-bearing and don't try to use big words (that is, polysyllabic circumlocutions or felicitous confabulations). You know the effect on you; they will have the same effect on the reader. Don't use big words, talk plainly. You'll be better appreciated.

Don't write from your viewpoint. Think about what the recipient of the letter might need or want, then he'll be more apt to read it. See the matter through the eyes of the reader.

Use fewer "I"s and more "you"s. Not "I want to thank you..." but "Thank you..." Not "I am requesting..." but "Please send me..." Even inject the name of the reader: "Please understand this letter, Charlie, because..."

Don't be insulting in a first letter. There are occasions when our anger gets the best of us—when someone has done something that seems to be despicable. But usually there are other considerations: this is a regular patient, this is a patient of a referring doctor, this is an insurance company that I want to have pay my bill. I really don't want to alienate them, even to win a point. So take it easy, be conciliatory in the first letter. As trite as the expression is, it says it best: You get more flies with honey than with vinegar. Plus, in most situations, there's enough time later for sarcasm and hostility (if that helps). And even then, if it's sarcastic or hostile, put it aside for at least a day or two before mailing it – you may change your mind.

Make it absolutely clear. Check carefully, whether while dictating or writing, and again before your letter goes out, to be sure your letter will be totally clear to the reader. You may understand it, but there can be many slips between conceiving, organizing, dictating, transcribing and typing. Don't take chances; be sure. Apply all the rules of good writing—be brief, be accurate and use no jargon, just to repeat a few.

Make it personal whenever possible. The more personal and friendly your letter, the better the acceptance of it. People will feel good reading it and be more favorably inclined to you, whatever your objective. Friendly does not necessarily mean jocular or overbearing or insincere. There is one caveat: If it is a hostile situation (on either side), friendliness is usually suspect and even may tend to be pandering. And the same goes for humor.

Make it neat. Letters prepared on a typewriter or computer are almost always neat. Only accidents, fluid spills, smearing of print, or torn envelopes, destroy neatness. But in the area of hand-written letters (and fortunately, they are fewer each year), it is easier to get sloppy. Neatness not only counts, it impresses.

Remember, you are responsible for your letters. Responsibility cannot be transferred to anyone else—a secretary, or an assistant. Alibis will not carry. Do it right the first time.

Preparing the Letter

Dates should be timely. The date on the letter should be the day it is typed. Be certain that the date is not too far from the occurrence. Seeing a patient in consultation on May 12 and dating the report on May 26 is too long a difference. Do your reports in a timely manner. Another gaffe is dating the letter July 14 and not getting around to mailing it (for whatever reason) until July 30. Be more efficient.

Be sure names and titles are absolutely correct. Both are important to the reader, and he or she would like to see them correct. It honors the person and will give the respect that his/her credentials earn. To address an optometrist as D.O. – or vice versa—means you don't care about his training, or his feelings — or don't understand the difference. If the reader has a title like President, Director, Dean, use it and limit your abbreviations.

Try to limit "Attention" lines. Whenever possible, address your letter directly to a person, by name. That recognizes him as a person or as an official. Never address a letter to "Squeedunk University" and then "Attention: President." Take the time to check out his name, or have someone do it. Usually, only a telephone call is necessary.

Use "Reference" line if possible. This line – usually located near the top of the page but below the name and address, near the right side --tells the reader immediately what the subject of the letter is, makes it easier for him to understand the communication, and makes it easier for both of you to file it or respond to it. It helps so much for the reader to know the name of the patient a medical report is about, or the subject of the correspondence in other letters.

Use first names in salutation, when acceptable. First, you must know the person. Then, you must know whether it is appropriate to address him by his first name. Personalities are different: some people love to be called by their first names; others holding official positions (and not knowing you well) may resent it.

When in doubt, use the formal greeting: Mr., Mrs., Miss, Ms., President, Dean, etc. When you use "Dr." as in "Dear Dr. Jones" it should be combined with using, in the address portion, the person's degree so that there is no misunderstanding of who he is:

John Jones, MD
1234 Front Street
Columbus, Ohio 12345

Dear Dr. Jones:

This clearly spells out the reader's occupation, and then salutes that person with proper respect. Using only the term "Dr." gives no specific information as to what profession is writing to what profession.

Don't use "hanging" closings. Examples are "With best regards, I am…" or the participle closing "Hoping to hear from you soon…" For older writers, that is a comfortable closing left over from their early days. Today it is not good form. Simply convert them to sentences, if you must use them, e.g., "I send my best regards" or "I hope to hear from you soon".

Make complimentary closings appropriate. While there is some movement to eliminate complimentary closings as redundant or outmoded, most of us will still continue to use them. Just make sure they are appropriate. A letter to your sister probably should not be signed "Sincerely", or a letter to your boss saying "Love." Still acceptable in appropriate spots are "Yours Truly," "Fraternally," "Respectfully" and others.

First name signatures. The rule here is easy. If you are on a first name basis, sign your first name only (even acceptable in legal controversies). If not, but you are willing to be addressed by your first name, or would like to be on a first name basis, sign with just your first name; it is an invitation.

Sign the letter yourself. No stamped signatures. No secretary signing your name and her initials. READ IT FIRST. If it is not satisfactory to you, rewrite it or retype it. After all, your signature authenticates everything in it.

Letters vs. other modes

So often the question comes up, "What is the best means of communicating?" There are some considerations that differentiate the use of various forms of communication. Briefly, the attributes of each are:

Letters. Use them when you want a written record, either for yourself, for the correspondent, for legal purposes, or so that a third party has evidence. Letters are good when there is no urgency, or limited urgency. With today's availability of overnight delivery, the urgency question is modified; it depends on when you want your correspondent to get the message. Cost is sometimes a consideration vis-a-vis other modes.

Telephone. This mode is quicker than letters, about equal to e-mail. It is less costly (The cost of producing a letter in an office runs several dollars.) On the other hand, if there is no urgency, a long letter to a foreign country is probably less expensive than a long telephone call. Depending on your purpose, it may be bad or good that there is no record of a telephone call (recording it is illegal without bilateral agreement). The only record of it may be the telephone company's records that it was made. When you don't want a written record, telephone is perfect.

e-mail. With regard to urgency, telephone and e-mail are about equal in timing, depending on whether your correspondent is immediately available. E-mail will give instantaneous transmission and leave your message even if the person is not in. It is fast, but there are problems with accuracy and permanence. There are no signatures giving authenticity. There will be a tendency to use computer jargon or e-mail slang, detracting from accuracy. In my opinion, the use of e-mails for important and "legal" information should be extremely limited, if used at all. Any such correspondence used in an emergency should be immediately followed up with a signed letter (perhaps return receipt requested).

In all these situations, good writing will make clearer what is happening and create less confusion among the participants.

REFERENCE

Freuhling, R.T., and Oldham, N.B.: *Write to the Point*! McGraw-Hill Book Company, 1988, 261 pages.

Chapter Eleven

Combative Letters
(Sample insurance case)

Many situations arise in our lives—both professional and personal—in which a combative letter may result, either ours or our correspondents. Writing well and carefully handling these letters will, many times, ease the tension, create more goodwill and possibly help solve the problem. Letters may be combative in attempting to right a wrong, or in replying to a combative or otherwise negative letter.

Because it illustrates so many principles involved, I shall devote this chapter to an exercise I have used in my Medical Writing classes. The insurance letter closely resembles many of the communications a health professional receives. My comments and recommendations are the result of examining the response letters written by hundreds of medical students, and is based on their mistakes.

The exercise

I gave each student a copy of a purported letter from an insurance company rejecting a claim, asking each one to write a reply as though he or she were the actual recipient of the letter. The results were amazing, mystifying, interesting, productive and illustrative. I read and analyzed every reply, codified them, noted common errors – and then drew certain conclusions. I found that the writing was excellent (better than for medical articles), but the communication was only fair. Some letters were exemplary, others…well!

In the rejection letter, I used, as bait to produce combative letters, the issue of recognition of osteopathic physicians and osteopathic manipulative therapy. After all, my students were going to become osteopathic physicians, and, even today, might still run into some discrimination. However, that does not change this discussion. Many other offensive rejections can occur: lack of certain qualifications, inadequate indications for a treatment or diagnosis, improper procedures and many other, even legitimate, rejections. The important fact is that there is a rejection, and the doctor becomes riled up.

Review of papers

Certain recurring comments or approaches were noted:

Failure to address correspondents accurately. Even though the letter was signed, a number of students addressed their letters to "Claims Manager" (with his name), or "Attention: Claims Manager" or "Dear Sir". One even said, "Dear Misinformed".

When a name is in the letter, address that person -- courteously. If you do not know to whom to address a letter of complaint, send it to the company president.

Insults. Many students immediately went to insults. Some of them were:

> Shed some light on your ignorance
> Relieve you of your ignorance
> As you should be aware
> Shocked and dismayed
> Enlighten you
> Bring your thinking into line

Insults and put-downs rarely solve problems. Tell your spouse but leave them out of your letters. Be assertive, but never lose your temper. You may act as though you might lose it, but once you do, the blame for the entire situation might get shifted to you. Belligerence and hostility, especially in a first letter, may be counter-productive.

Re-submitting the bill. Why bother? They already have it, have analyzed it and have responded to it. They don't need another bill. Make your case, instead.

Demeaning others. " I am better able to manage such cases." "My training is better than most doctors." Although this was not a frequent finding, it still is meaningless to demean others to advance your point – and it gains you nothing.

Threats. Included were threats to take legal action, file suit, or go to the insurance commissioner. First, these are empty threats if you don't know what you are talking about. Are you sure that you have a legitimate legal case? Do you know for sure that this is something that violates the insurance commissioner's rules, or the state's? Don't threaten if you are not sure. Then there's the practical point: Most insurance companies have staffs of attorneys working full time on nothing but insurance cases—so they are hardly likely to be intimidated by your threats. They also know that most threats to sue are empty and are never carried out. On the other hand, if you feel strongly that you have an appropriate legal standing, CONSULT YOUR LAWYER! And do it before you send that threat.

Referring the company to an official agency. Used were agencies such as the State Board of Examiners, the State Association, the national organization. But...but, *you* do it for them! You are the one who wants to get some money or prove a point. They won't do the searching or inquiring; you must do it for them – and produce the results -- to convince them. If you are sure you are covered by an agency, don't refer the reader to it. Simply send a copy of your letter to that agency and indicate it at the bottom of your letter.

Referring to state law or statutes or rules. Some of the students made this reference without knowing whether such regulations existed or they applied. Do not refer to official documents unless you are sure they exist and apply to your case. Certainly an insurance company (or other institution) is more likely to know all those regulations than you are. Check first if you are not absolutely positive.

"Do not hesitate to call me." A few students included a conciliatory line like that – a great idea! It's always good to leave the door open to further communication.

Discussion

With all the variants that appeared, a strong consideration of guidelines is and was in order.

First of all, the letter writer should decide in advance the objective of his letter. Most of the time, the objective is to succeed in your claim—to collect the money, to be approved, to have a claim settled or a number of possible other goals.

Once you have chosen your objective, keep your eye upon the doughnut and not upon the hole! Do everything needed to achieve your goal, do not deviate to secondary objectives. Among secondary objectives which usually get in the way of reaching the primary goal are:

Revenge

Express hostility

Salving hurt feelings

A wise lawyer once told me, "Get the money first and worry about the satisfaction afterward." I have never forgotten that and it has always been right. Doughnut again.

One objective that may arise is mid-way between these two. There may be an objective to protect or defend your profession (substitute as needed: hospital, reputation, type of practice or whatever) because of something in the offensive letter. The defense should not be emotional, but factual. Quote—or even send them publications –from official bodies, legislatures, courts, and make your defense strong with them.

Conclusion

At the end of every exercise, students would ask me, "What would you do? How would you answer the letter?" Let me count the ways:

1. I would carefully try to discover why the claim was rejected. Solving the problem is easier than fighting. Was there some sort of misunderstanding among me, the insurance company and the patient? I would look first at my role in it. Was there anything not clear about my billing? About the diagnosis? About the charge? About the indication for a procedure? Was the billing (or diagnosis or treatment) against the company policy and I did not know it?

2. Having examined my own part in the controversy, and finding nothing, I would then try to determine whether the reviewer was not aware of something in the medical aspect of the case or the insurance aspect. I would follow up on that.

3. I would then answer the letter gently. Maybe even write, "I really hate to say anything, but…" [1] I would explain what I did medically or surgically, and go far beyond the usual filling in the blanks. I would explain the osteopathic

profession (or the comparable objection) and send information about osteopathic medicine (or my credentials or my hospital or whatever). I would explain the medical status of the patient completely and thoroughly and clearly. Then I would ask for a review of the claim.

4. If I did not succeed, I would draft a strong letter, with firmer language, maybe with an implied threat, but no specifics, e.g., " I have given you every opportunity to settle this matter but if we cannot reach an agreement, I may be forced to follow other avenues to achieve my objective." Sometimes it is wise to sprinkle the words "shocked", "appalled", "dismayed" or even " outrageous and horrific", especially in the first sentence (1).

5. My third letter would be the hammer. I would make threats that I knew to be correct and could be supported (not just idle ones), whether legal suit, invoking the Secretary of Health or advising other agencies or whatever is applicable. However, I would first call my lawyer and ask his opinion. Being firm does not means being reckless, and I must protect myself as well as seek conclusion of the matter to my satisfaction.

Always remember the two hackneyed aphorisms, as they are so applicable: "You get more flies with honey than with vinegar" and "Keep you eye on the doughnut and not on the hole."

Throughout all this letter writing and, in addition to the strategies, never lose sight of the important fact that good writing makes for more understanding between combatants, that good grammar may convince more than poor grammar, and that poor punctuation may scuttle the intent of your letters. These are not matters — whether with insurance companies, governmental agencies, lawyers or patients –- that can be dismissed lightly. Protect your reputation and your interests with every means possible.

REFERENCE

1. Phillips, Ellen: *Shocked, Appalled and Dismayed! How to Write Letters of Complaint That Get Results.* Vantage Books, 1999, 333pages. Quoted in USA Today, September 12, 2000.

Bibliography

I am indebted to the authors listed below for what I have garnered from their writings, and for the opportunity to know them, and learn directly from them:

Godden, J.O.: Mind to Mind: Persuasion in Medical Writing. Canadian Medical Association Journal, April 1, 1967, p. 953-964.

Godden, J.O.: Maxims to Help Aspiring Physician-Writers Get Started. Canadian Family Physician, January 1973.

Huth, E.J.: How to Write and Publish Papers in the Medical Sciences, 2nd edition. Baltimore. Williams and Wilkins, 1996.

Huth, E.J.: Medical Style and Format: An International Manual for Authors, Editors, and Publishers.

Philadelphia. Institute for Scientific Information Press, 1987.

King, Lester S. and Roland, Charles G. : Scientific Writing. Chicago. American Medical Association, 1968.

Peterson, Barbara: Basic Medical Writing. Chicago. American Osteopathic Association, 1965.

Schwager, Edith: Medical English Usage and Abusage. Phoenix. Oryx Press, 1991.

Schwager, Edith, Editor: On Medical Communications. Bethesda. American Medical Writers Association, 1982.

Recommended Readings

Bernstein, T.M.: The Careful Writer: A Modern Guide to English Usage. New York. Atheneum, 1967.

Burchfield, R.W.: The New Fowler's Modern English Usage. Oxford. Clarendon Press. 1996.

Hewitt, Richard M.: The Physician-Writer's Book: Tricks of the Trade of Medical Writing. Philadelphia. W.B. Saunders Company, 1957.

Merriam-Webster's Manual for Writers and Editors. Springfield. Merriam-Webster, 1998.

Minick, Phyllis, Editor: Biomedical Communication: Selected AMWA Workshops. Bethesda. American Medical Writers Association, 1994.

O'Conner, Patricia T.: Words Fail Me: What Everyone Who Writes Should Know About Writing. New York. Harcourt Brace & Company, 1999.

O'Conner, Patricia T.: Woe Is I: The Grammarphobe's Guide to Better English in Plain English. New York. Riverhead Books, 1996

Saltzman, Joel: If You Can Talk, You Can Write. New York. Warner Books, 1993.

Strunk, William, Jr., and White, E.B.: The Elements of Style, 3rd edition. New York. Macmillan Publishing Company, 1979

Zinsser, William K.: On Writing Well, 6th edition. New York. HarperPerennial, 1998.

Reference Books

Any standard dictionary, especially Webter's Collegiate.

Oxford English Dictionary. Oxford. Oxford University Press, 1971.

Roget's Thesaurus – any edition

Made in the USA
Monee, IL
11 February 2020